ABOUT T

Tales from The Bedside is a collection of true sto...

experiences as a Critical Care Registered Nurse. I've been an RN for twenty-plus years and I've been working the night shift for as long as I've had my nursing license. I love the night shift! I received my RN degree in 1992 from the College of Central Florida. I took rigorous critical-care training in 1998 at Munroe Regional Medical Center, a prestigious magnet hospital in Florida. The mentorship and extensive training I received there are priceless. I'm grateful beyond measure for the generosity of those I've trained and worked with.

ICU nursing is beyond compare. Yes, it's a never-a-dull-moment ride. I've seen, done, heard, and experienced the best of the best! I will never stop learning. And I've been extremely fortunate to have traveled the country. I've practiced in several cities, in multiple states including Florida, Maryland, Utah, and Colorado. I've worked in rural hospitals, big teaching hospitals, and level-one trauma centers. My specialty is adult critical care and the majority of my nursing experience has been in critical care, but my experience is vast. I've worked in Oncology, Telemetry, Urology Clinic,

Cardiovascular Step Down, Emergency, and Adult Critical Care: ICU, CCU, MICU, CVICU, SICU, and PACU.

I'm a hardcore patient advocate. I will not hesitate to speak up on behalf of my patients in order to keep them safe and well cared for. My vast nursing experience, critical thinking skills, outstanding work ethic, and caring attitude greatly benefit my patients, I like to think. Their safety and wellbeing are my top priority when I'm in the workplace. Remember this … when you think that we don't care, we do.

My hope is to enlighten you as to what goes on behind the scenes. My stories do not contain the real names of the patients and facilities, but they are real stories.

I'm also a hobby photographer. I captured my cover photo on one of my hiking adventures in Utah. Fitness and healthy living are very important to me. One of my favorite exercises is hiking the great outdoors. I post my photos and never-ending adventure stories on Instagram, Twitter, and Facebook. I also have an endearing habit of referring to myself as SK in all of my stories.

Thank you for letting me share. Happy reading, everyone!

RECTAL TUBE

It was one of those nights in the dungeon, aka ICU. We were extremely busy. I'm accustomed to hearing all sorts of sounds from patients, monitors, equipment, my coworkers, etc. One elderly patient was very confused. He was having delusions and hallucinations. He was also excreting severe liquid diarrhea due to an intestinal bacteria called C-difficile toxin.

C-diff is a spore that is highly contagious. We had to contain his stools to prevent the spread of infection. Rectal tube to the rescue! I don't think it's necessary for me to describe in detail how we insert it. Yes, we use a generous amount of lubricant, but still I felt really bad for the patient as he screamed "Rape!" during the procedure.

Sad.

FOLEY

He was obnoxious. I can't think of any other word to describe him. Well, I can, but I won't utter it. He was our "town special" for the night, going through severe alcohol withdrawals. I had given him enough benzos to kill an elephant, yet he continued to scream profanity, be combative, and just plain disgusting. He called me terrible names. He was beyond reason. We had to put him in a full body restraint.

Oh yes, ER and ICU nurses know how to tie your ass down. The full body restraint literally keeps a highly combative patient in place. It's a lifesaver. Without it, we risk serious injury to our hospital staff. Once the patient was secure, I calmly told him that I needed to insert a Foley catheter. A Foley catheter ensures accurate urine output measurement in an incontinent, sedated, or critically ill patient. He was all of the above.

I told the patient the following: "The Foley catheter goes through your penis and into your bladder. Upon insertion, I will inflate the balloon at the tip of the catheter to keep the Foley in place. Any attempts to tug or pull the Foley may result in urethral trauma—

including bleeding, severe pain, swelling, and loss of penile erection. If you value your penis, you will stay silent and listen to me."

He immediately stopped fighting and screaming, then he said something that made me feel very sorry for him.

"Please don't do that. I promise to be good. Please … please …"

While he begged, I continued to prepare my Foley insertion kit, prepped his meatus, and inserted the Foley catheter without any difficulty.

Winner.

CLUMSY

I've dropped my patient's stool softener on the floor twice when I went to open it. So I have to go back to the Pyxis three times to get one.

My patient is such a gentleman, though. He says that third time's the charm. I'm just silently saying *WTF* about my clumsiness. LOL!

I expect the pharmacist to come marching into the ICU at change of shift. I better try to act remorseful.

FREQUENT FLYER

She's a "frequent flyer" in our hospital. She suffers from chronic lung disease, as a result of years of heavy cigarette smoking. She's been here many times due to respiratory failure, often requiring a ventilator.

Wikipedia: *A mechanical ventilator is a machine designed to move breathable air into and out of the lungs, to provide breathing for a patient who is physically unable to breathe, or breathing insufficiently.*

Tonight is just like the others. She presented to my ICU in severe respiratory distress. She had deep, labored breathing and she was using all of her accessory muscles to breathe. She was only able to speak in very short sentences. I knew right away that we would be intubating and putting her on a ventilator soon. Before I could even put the heart monitor on her, she asked if she could go outside to smoke. Imagine that.

Shortly thereafter, we intubated her and put her on the ventilator. Just like the previous admissions, we had been unable to wean her off the ventilator, so we shipped her to a higher level of care for more specialized pulmonary management.

Will I see her again? Well, the body can only put up with so much abuse.

Sad but true.

TIME-OUT

She was my last patient in PACU. She did very well after surgery. We had been waiting for a bed assignment for over an hour. While we waited, she regaled me with stories about her life, her beloved horses, and her hospital-setting experiences as a patient. She told me of an experience that had me in stitches.

Once upon a time, she was rushed to the ER after falling off a horse. Her left leg was extremely swollen and painful. Her leg x-ray showed a leg fracture. She was immediately prepped for surgery. The OR crew came to transport her and the OR nurse said, "We're going to fix your appendix."

Feeling alarmed, the patient responded, "There's nothing wrong with my appendix. I need surgery on my left leg." The nurse disagreed and even reassured the patient that she wouldn't be feeling pain anytime soon. The patient, on the verge of a panic attack, insisted on talking to the trauma surgeon to whom she gave informed consent earlier. The nurse responded by saying that time was of the essence, that they had to hurry. At this point, the patient, now full-blown panic mode, started screaming and demanded to see the doctor ... "NOW!"

The ER doctor who saw the patient earlier came to her rescue. He pulled back the thin sheet covering the patient's legs and told the nurse to go back to nursing school.

MULTITASKING GONE BAD

It was one of those nights. We hit the floor, running. I never stopped unless I had to empty my bladder. At one point, I noticed my colleague frantically calling the other units asking the same question: "Do you have it?"

Apparently, he hit the *empty send* button on the tube system when he meant to hit the *lab* button to send the blood specimens that he drew from his patient. The *empty send* button will drop the tube system container anywhere in the hospital where a tube container is needed.

I didn't have time to find out whether he found his specimens or not.

What a night!

HOLY SMOKES

Once upon a time, I was busy charting on my ICU patients when I heard a rapid-response called overhead. The rapid-response was initiated by the floor nursing staff because a patient needed immediate assistance beyond the capability of the current staff. Sometimes, they transfer the patient to ICU, depending on the severity or nature of the emergency.

Apparently, the nursing staff on the floor smelled smoke. They immediately searched the area. It led them to a patient's room. They witnessed the patient in his hospital bed frantically trying to put out a small fire around him. He was still wearing his oxygen via nasal cannula. His face and hands were charred from the fiery explosion he caused when he lit up a cigarette.

CRITICAL-CARE INSTINCT

A lady in her forties came to our rural ER for persistent nausea and vomiting. She was given IVF for dehydration and antiemetic for nausea, then sent home. She came back to the ER later that night with worsened nausea. This time, they did a cardiac workup. Her twelve-lead EKG showed ST changes, but her cardiac enzymes were normal. She denied chest discomfort.

Based on these findings, she was admitted to the medical–surgical floor for further observation. There, she had tachycardia (elevated heart rate) and continued nausea. By early morning, I was notified that they needed to transfer this patient to my ICU because she was now hypertensive and needed IV medications.

When I received her, the patient's chief complaint was severe nausea. She denied chest pain. Despite the absence of chest discomfort, I immediately recognized the signs and symptoms of an active myocardial infarction (heart attack): pallor, severe malaise, cold sweats, flu-like symptoms, hypertension, and tachycardia. I immediately put oxygen on her and gave her medications to lower her blood pressure and heart rate. I also followed my rule to always advocate for my patients. I calmly told the Hospitalist MD who was sitting at the nursing station, "The patient is having a heart attack. She needs to be transferred to a higher level of care right away or she'll die."

The MD listened to me. We immediately summoned the flight team to transport the patient to a level-one trauma center, whose cardiac cath team, eagerly awaiting the patient, took her directly to the cath lab upon arrival. I was later informed that the patient had a severe blockage of the left main artery in her heart. We call that type of blockage, the "widow maker." They placed her on an intra-aortic balloon pump (IABP) to rest her heart before undergoing an open-heart bypass surgery shortly thereafter.

PATIENT DELIGHT

My patient who is seventy-seven years young is such a delight! She loves telling stories of her only daughter and her pets. She happened to fall in love with me. LOL.

Patient: "I wish I was built like you. What nationality are you? I was telling my husband how gorgeous you are. You should be a model."

SK: "Thank you! I'm a model. I'm Filipino."

Patient: "Is that the same as Japanese?"

SK: "No, totally different but we're both Asians."

Patient: "I used to be a beautiful shit. People couldn't tell my age."

SK: "You still are! You just don't feel well, so you naturally feel like you don't look your best."

Patient: "I'm gonna call home to talk to my dogs. They miss me so much."

She proceeded to tell me how her dogs talk to her. She was a hoot!

The day-shift male RN would not be excluded. Here's how Kurtis spent his day with our lovely patient. Kurtis accompanied the patient during her walk in the hospital hallways.

Patient: "I can't believe I brought this old robe. Early in our marriage, my husband bought me some lingerie. My boobs were too small for it. That's okay. My husband said that anything over a mouthful is a waste."

Kurtis said he was dying … and was sure blushing! LOL.

CONFUSED NOT

Once upon a night, I was floated to the medical surgical unit. I received a report on a ninety-one-year-old gentleman. I was told that he had severe dementia and was very confused. His son stayed with him at night.

After receiving the report, I went to see him. He was alone and resting quietly in bed. I introduced myself and flashed him my most charming smile. He looked at me with alert eyes, smiled and said, "You're cute!"

What was my nursing assessment? The patient was alert and oriented (*wink!*).

JEKYLL and HYDE

It was my lucky night. I received a report from the ER about a patient who was brought in for alcohol intoxication. He was sedated and on a ventilator. I was told to count my blessings.

Just a few hours ago, my patient was not the calm, sleeping teddy bear I initially laid eyes on. His neighbors called 911 when they heard him pounding on their door and noticed his drunken state. Police officers and emergency medical services responded. While they were loading him into the back of the ambulance, the patient became belligerent and punched one of the paramedics on the face. Huge mistake!

The rescue squad arrived in the ER with a severely combative patient who was in four-point restraints—handcuffs around his wrists and shackles around his ankles, secured to the stretcher rails. The ER personnel, who I love for their no-nonsense ways, immediately sedated, paralyzed, and intubated the patient.

The plan was to let his alcohol level return to normal, turn off his sedation, and extubate him once he passed the spontaneous breathing trial. I was also instructed to call the police officers before we turned off the patient's sedation. They wanted to be present when the patient woke up.

Everything went smoothly with the extubation process. There were three police officers at the patient's bedside. The patient was alert, oriented, and cooperative. One of my colleagues who knew the patient personally had informed me earlier that the patient was a high-functioning alcoholic and one of the nicest guys you could ever meet. He was a devoted father, had a good-paying job, and was a good citizen. His drinking problem had escalated after his wife decided to file for divorce.

The patient was extremely remorseful when he learned about what he did. He claimed that he didn't remember anything. Fortunately, the people in this small town, including the paramedic he punched, knew him well enough to believe him and forgive him. No charges were filed.

HEAVEN SENT

I was assessing my patient's neurological status.

SK: "Tell me where you are"

Patient: "In heaven," he said … followed by a radiant smile and a wink.

SK: "I love my job!"

LET ME GO

He had end-stage lung disease. He had been in the hospital for over a month. He would get better, warranting transfer from the ICU to the regular floor. He made it two days on the floor before transferring back to ICU due to increased respiratory distress. He had multiple comorbidities. I took care of him for many nights. With each passing night, his condition worsened. His doctors gave him a very poor prognosis. They also discussed end-of-life options, including hospice. Hospice allows us to provide comfort and dignity to a terminally ill patient. Once the patient and family choose hospice, we stop all heroic measures—no more painful interventions, no more unnecessary patient suffering. We provide care and support for the patient and the entire family. We give medications generously to ease the patient's suffering.

He did not want heroic measures performed if he stopped breathing or if his heart stopped. However, his wife felt differently. She wanted to keep him alive at all costs. He wanted to honor her wishes more than his own, so he chose to be Full Code (full life-saving measures). His current wife and his daughters from a previous marriage despised each other. Having had the opportunity to watch their family dynamics, I came to the conclusion that his children would honor his wishes more than their own. He had been able to direct his own care, but he was almost out of time.

He was well on his way to multi-organ system failure. He was in kidney failure requiring dialysis, ischemic heart failure, and end-stage lung disease. He required a BIPAP mask at high settings. He was extremely claustrophobic, so he could only wear the BIPAP mask for a few hours before he ripped it off. He became angry and belligerent when we explained the importance of keeping the mask on. When he continued to refuse, his breathing worsened. He was in constant air hunger. Yet, he continued to refuse the one life-saving device that would help him rest—the ventilator. The ventilator is a machine that breathes for you. He knew that choosing the ventilator would only prolong his agony. To him, it meant that he would spend the rest of his life in a long-term care facility, strapped to a breathing machine.

The nights were agonizing for him and for his daughters, who took turns staying with him at night. His wife stayed with him each day. I watched him fight a war that he would ultimately lose. One night, I was at his bedside, securing the BIPAP mask that he ripped off for the tenth time, when he exclaimed, "I'm dying. I want to go home." It was a heart-wrenching moment that I will never forget.

I held his hand and thanked him for the privilege of caring for him. I told him that I would keep him and his family in my prayers. He thanked me and gave me his most heartwarming smile. He always called me by name, even through his delirium. He never failed to thank me for keeping him clean and comfortable. He passed away later that day. He died peacefully and pain free, surrounded by his loving family.

Rest in peace, my dear one. You will always hold a special place in my heart.

OH, THE NERVE

I could feel the energy in the air. It would be a night to remember.

I noticed a commotion at the end of the hallway. Doctors, nurses, supervisors, hospital security guards, and police officers congregated in front of Room 7. They all had that *WTF*-look clearly plastered on their faces. I've always been a curious spirit, so I went to inquire about the situation. The patient's nurse told me what happened.

The patient had apparently hidden a bag of crack cocaine and a lighter in his underwear. He just arrived in ICU and the night shift just came on. The night-shift nurse assessed the patient, then walked out to get his medications for the night. When she returned, there was a cloud of smoke in the room. The patient, who had just inhaled his fix, was frantically trying to hide the proof of his deed.

The nurse became immediately ill upon inhaling the smoke. She was nauseous all night from inhaling the fumes. The patient earned a 1:1 guard. He went to jail upon discharge from the hospital.

Patients like him put everyone in the hospital in danger. A hospital room can be turned into a massive bomb when fire is introduced. It's an oxygen rich environment. What happens when fire and oxygen mix?

Exactly.

.

FIRE HAZARD

My patient is a lovely elderly lady. Despite her multiple health problems and current condition, she has maintained her sense of humor. I assisted her with her PM care (bed bath, oral care) and assisted her to the reclining chair. While I was changing her bed linens, she asked if there was anything I could give her to moisturize her lips. I saw a container of lip cream on her table, so I handed it to her. The lip product is provided by our hospital facility for our patients.

She proceeded to tell me that one of the nurses told her to never use it around oxygen because it might cause a fire. She used oxygen via nasal cannula. I explained to her that all of our hospital products we used for our patients were safe to use. The lip moisturizer was not petroleum based. Petroleum-based products are discouraged because it's considered to be highly flammable in the presence of oxygen.

She trusted my information. I allayed her fears and she had moist lips to boot! She ended our conversation by saying, "Well, I guess if I blow myself up, I'm in the right place."

Oh my …

SHIT HITS THE FAN

She weighed 350+ pounds. She had sustained multiple crushing injuries and a flail chest from a motor-vehicle accident. She was on the ventilator, sedated, and receiving continuous feeding of a liquid formula through a nasogastric tube. She had not had a bowel movement in days. Yes, it was just a matter of time before the inevitable happened.

The first phase happened on my shift. She "gave birth," to say the least. It took four people and over two hours to maneuver through the mess. Every time we turned the patient on her side to clean her back and change her bed linens, her oxygen saturation (SAO2) would go down below 90% very quickly. Her ventilator settings were at maximum and delivering 100% FIO2. Every time her SAO2 dropped, we would roll her to a supine position, elevate the head of the bed, and let the ventilator do its thing until her SAO2 were above 90%. Every time we rolled her back and forth, she rewarded us with massive amounts of flatus and stool. It was a never-ending *shitstorm*. The massive amount of stool she was producing throughout this show, evolved from solid to loose to liquid, so in the end, we had to insert a rectal tube … which is a whole other story. LMAO.

Needless to say, she was clean and comfortable after it was all over. The day shift would not be spared. The rectal tube leaked (as most rectal tubes do), so the nurses decided that it was a good time to give her a bed bath. When they turned the patient on her side, she literally exploded from her butt. Liquid diarrhea, propelled by massive flatus, flew from her butt, hitting the nurses, the walls, the curtain, and the windows.

Holy shit, indeed.

CODE BLUE

Call it gut instinct. Upon assessing my patient, I had this feeling that something was going to happen that night. The patient was admitted earlier during the day for chest pain. His cardiac workup was unremarkable, but we were doing serial cardiac markers by drawing his blood every four hours to check for elevation of cardiac enzymes. Cardiac markers are used to evaluate heart function. He was chest-pain free when I assessed him and his vital signs were stable.

An hour went by when I noticed that his heart rate went from 70s (normal sinus rhythm) to 50s (sinus bradycardia); he was feeling weak but nothing unusual, his blood pressure stable, skin warm and dry. The feeling of dread continued, so I immediately went to the nursing station and informed everyone to prepare for a code blue. I explained the patient's symptoms. I received curious stares from everyone, so I told them that I had this gut feeling. Sure enough, within fifteen minutes of my announcement, the patient's heart rate slowed down drastically, eventually going into asystole. We immediately called a code blue and went to work to save his life. We tried all of the life-saving techniques and medications for as long as we could. The patient never recovered despite our heroic measures.

The MD who was running the code finally called it, and then he asked me to give the dead patient some Morphine IV. I was perplexed as to why I would give a dead patient pain medicine. He explained that it was the least we could do for him after we pumped on his chest, inserted tubes in his body, and shot electrical current through his heart. His very kind gesture and professionalism touched my heart.

We care ... very much.

FREQUENT-FLYER PROGRAM

She was one of our frequent flyers. Someone who must have cared a little about her called 911 when they found her unresponsive. A twenty-something female diagnosed with type-1 diabetes when she was a child, she had been very noncompliant with her care, preferring to indulge in recreational drugs. It was her perfect way to escape reality. She hadn't been checking her blood sugars at home nor had she taken any of her long- and short-acting insulin. She was in severe diabetic ketoacidosis (DKA).

She was quite somnolent when I admitted her to ICU. She was positive for illegal drugs in her toxicology screen (no surprises there). She was on the DKA protocol and was responding quite well. The DKA treatment protocol consists of insulin drip, IV fluid boluses, IV fluids with electrolytes, frequent blood-sugar checks, and serial lab tests. We continue this intensive treatment until the patient is out of DKA. The patient pretty much slept throughout the night shift and I gave a report to the day-shift nurse.

When I came back the following night, I went to check on my assignment that was posted on the wall. That's when I saw the patient, looking alive and well, dash through the double doors, never to be seen again. At least up till now.

Apparently, once she was out of DKA and became alert and oriented, she demanded to go home. She became extremely angry when she realized that the bag of marijuana she had with her when she came in had been confiscated by security and disposed of properly. She screamed all sorts of profanity at the nurses. She got dressed, took out her own IVs, and walked out the door. No thank-you notes, of course.

Who pays for her hospital bill? We (tax payers, the hospital) do.

911

A 911 dispatcher calls to inform us that a patient in our unit called 911. When the dispatcher asked the patient, "What is your emergency?" the patient replied, "They're trying to kill me." The patient was very confused, hallucinating, and delusional. The patient, who had underlying psych issues, was admitted for polysubstance overdose.

This is not an uncommon occurrence. I've seen this scene played many times across the board. The same scenario with ever-changing characters.

'TIS THE SEASON

A patient in his early forties who came into the ER tonight in a severely critical condition was flown to a higher level of care due to pneumonia complications. This particular patient is also diabetic with uncontrolled blood sugar levels and has multiple comorbidities that contribute to his severe condition.

A CT scan of his chest showed air bubbles all the way up his left lung. Meaning, bacteria is festering and he'll need a thoracotomy (open lung surgery) to remove the infected part of his lung. Which needs to be done ASAP. He's facing long hospital stay and extensive antibiotic therapy—among other things.

My point:

1) People with pre-existing medical conditions such as asthma or diabetes, the very young, or elderly are at higher risk of acquiring pneumonia. Don't wait too long to see your doctor or go to the hospital.

2) If you're diabetic, keep your blood sugar under control. Easier said than done, but if you want to live a quality life, it's a must. And stop smoking. Seriously!

3) Wash your hands frequently. HAND WASHING is the single most important step in preventing the spread of infection. Hand sanitizers are a great alternative if you don't have immediate access to soap and water.

A DAY in the LIFE of an ALCOHOLIC

Once upon a time, I admitted a patient with severe alcohol intoxication with suicidal ideation. He had been drinking vodka all day. His wife called 911 when he threatened to kill a doctor and commit suicide by having police officers shoot him to death. He had a long history of alcohol abuse. He started drinking at thirteen years old. He was mid-thirties when I had him as a patient.

He was given a very strong sedative/anti-psychotic in the ER because he was combative, though by the time I assumed care of him in ICU, he was calm and cooperative. When I walked into his room, I addressed him by his name and introduced myself. He immediately showered me with compliments and called me a sweetheart. At that point, I knew we would get along just fine. LOL.

That said, I had to remind him of his manners several times, but I managed to knock him out with some powerful benzos. Twelve hours later, with his alcohol level down to a normal level, he was a completely different man—subdued, withdrawn, and depressed. I consider people like him "wasted talent." Alcoholism is a national epidemic.

FACT: alcohol addiction can cause multi-organ system failure—including the brain. It has serious ramifications on your family life and social life. In other words, *it sucks the life out of you*. And it brings down others with you.

HEROIN

He was a thirty-one-year-old guy who had been shooting up heroin for five years. He was admitted to my ICU for septic shock (secondary to shooting up a bad batch of heroin in his vein). His blood pressure was dangerously low, so he was started on vasoactive drip and IV fluids via a central venous line in his right intra-jugular vein. His toxicology screen was also positive for opiates, cannabis, and amphetamines. Soon, he was suffering from withdrawal symptoms (pain, agitation, restlessness).

Nothing we did to alleviate his suffering was good enough for him. Unbeknownst to us, he called up his drug-dealing friend.

Fast forward to the day shift. Per the patient's request, he was assisted to the bathroom and provided privacy. When he was finished, he was assisted back in bed. The brilliant day-shift ICU RN noticed that his demeanor seemed unusually calmer … and he had a sock missing from his right foot.

When she looked closely, she saw the top of his right foot was bleeding. Soon after, he was surrounded by the MD, charge nurse, and the primary care RN. After thorough questioning, the patient admitted to shooting up heroin through his right foot vein while he was in the bathroom. Fortunately, the patient was NOT smart enough to use his central line to inject his drug of choice that his so-called friend brought for him. Hospital security found the syringe he used, wrapped in a paper towel in the trash can.

The local police officers came. His friend, who had several outstanding warrants, was arrested. The patient was suffering from multiple comorbidities due to his chronic IV drug use, but still his mother continued to enable her son's behavior and addiction. She had threatened the healthcare staff with negative consequences if her son did not feel better soon. Never mind that her son received top-notch care from one of the most proficient, highly skilled, caring healthcare providers in the nation.

THIS is the reality we sometimes face: being unappreciated, hated, threatened, verbally and physically abused. Why do I choose ICU nursing?

Sometimes, I really don't know. I just do.

PAIN

Nursing 101: Pain Is Subjective

When a patient complains of pain and requests pain medicine, your duty as a nurse is to assess the type, source, degree, and the associated symptoms of the pain, and then provide the appropriate pain relief. If pain medicine has already been ordered, you give it. If pain medicine has not been ordered, you get an order from the MD.

We were taught in nursing school that pain is subjective. You need to disregard your personal biases and never impose your own judgment on your patient. Don't withhold pain medication based on your personal biases. Ever.

I've had altercations with fellow nurses and physicians because pain medicine was withheld or not ordered, based on their personal biases. My colleagues who know me well and have witnessed these events have said that they would NOT dare provoke me to wear my boxing gloves. Ever. LOL.

I'm a hardcore patient advocate. Period.

I recognize drug seeking behavior when I see it. I also recognize when my patient truly needs pain medication. In both cases, I provide the best possible care and education I'm capable of giving.

The following story will hopefully help you understand why I'm passionate about pain management.

I admitted a patient who was a known IV drug user. She had shot heroin in her right arm, using a non-sterile needle. Within a few hours, she was in full-blown sepsis. She was severely hypotensive requiring a vasoactive drip. Her right arm was very swollen and looked extremely painful. She was clearly in pain. Her pain was properly managed with an adequate combination of pain medications. She verbalized being satisfied with our pain management.

I gave a report to the day-shift crew, feeling good about the care I'd provided my patient that night. When I came back the following night, my patient was in severe distress due to pain. Apparently, an MD who has a reputation for being difficult—and who, I believe, harbors this idea that drug addicts should suffer the consequences of their actions—discontinued the IV pain medication and reduced the PO (by mouth) pain medication, both of which were helping the patient stay fairly comfortable. The patient was writhing in pain when I saw her and her right arm was even more swollen. I was not happy, to say the least. I immediately paged the MD responsible for the patient's suffering. She showed up. I explained to her about the patient's condition. I requested to have the original pain medication-combo resumed. She refused and gave me the most idiotic reason for not doing so.

We exchanged words and I bluntly told her that she didn't belong in critical care. By the grace of God, the oncoming night-shift MD came to the rescue. He resumed the proper combination of pain medications, which eased the patient's suffering. The following day, a surgeon who was consulted to evaluate the affected arm recommended surgery right away. The increased swelling caused "compartment syndrome." Compartment syndrome is a medical emergency that requires immediate surgery. Without surgical intervention, the patient would have lost her arm or worse, her life. She was immediately flown to a higher level of care for emergency surgical intervention.

Relief swept over me.

WHY OH WHY?

He's African American. He has severe mental illness. He was in our ER because he cut off his penis. When asked why he did that. He said that he wanted a "white penis."

Why. Oh. Why …?

WOE IS ME

He's four hundred-plus pounds, resigned to a life of immobility, and plagued with comorbidities of his own contriving. He's been in our hospital for over a month, shuffling between ICU, the rehab unit, and the skilled nursing unit. Today, he's back in our ICU with acute coronary syndrome. His cardiac catheterization showed three-vessel disease. The interventional cardiologist was unable to open and stent the blockages. The only option was open heart surgery.

He was initially deemed too unstable for open heart surgery due to his current medical condition: morbid obesity, pulmonary edema, and chronic tracheostomy due to chronic respiratory failure. Furthermore, he has been very noncompliant with his care. He refuses to get out of bed for his physical therapy, refuses to be turned or repositioned in bed, and refuses bed baths because he can't tolerate having the head of the bed lowered. The only thing he has been enjoying is indulging in two trays of food for each meal while on the regular floors. Once back in ICU, his diet was changed to an eighteen-hundred-calorie, cardiac diet. Guess who received the brunt of his wrath?

Yes, he was eventually cleared for open heart surgery. When the charge RN went to give his pre-operative education, he flatly refused to listen, telling her bluntly, "I don't want to hear about it!"

How did he do after surgery? Honestly, there are times when we can't always find it in ourselves to care as much as at other times.

THE LIE

Once upon a time, I took care of a patient who came in for some unexplained chest pain and shortness of breath. We did extensive testing to find out what was wrong with him. We were prepared to do more. When his urine toxicology screen came back, it was positive for cocaine. When I asked him if he'd smoked anything or snorted anything, he lied and said he hadn't.

I told him that his urine toxicology screen came back positive for cocaine. Looking embarrassed, he continued to lie. He said that he was with his friends who were smoking cocaine. Apparently, he was cooped up in the same room with them for three hours. I told him that he would have had to ingest the cocaine himself for it to be in his system. I also told him to never lie to us because it could save his life. It's also a waste of resources, time, and energy. And, I can't help it, but it pisses the shit out of me.

Tell the TRUTH, no matter what. Lying is for cowards.

Rant over.

PARENTS' LOVE

I was a witness to the pure, unconditional love of a mother and a father. A love for a son who had completely lost himself to alcohol. A severe alcohol withdrawal brings out one's darkest side.

Best part of my night? Being told "Yes, Mommy," by my patient who thought I was as bossy as his mom. LOL.

FAREWELL

He touched my heart. I held his hand before I left this morning. I told him that it had been an honor to take care of him. Even through his delirium at night, he always called me by my name. He always managed to say thank you and smiled when he could. My RN friend who took care of him on day shift told me that he spoke so nicely about me. He looked forward to seeing me every time I came on shift.

My dearest patient died peacefully that day I said my last goodbye. I took care of him for many nights.

He was a gentle warrior. His memory lives on …

VETERANS: I HONOR THEM

Some of my cherished memories in my nursing career involve caring for veterans. A lot of them served their time in my home country, the Philippines.

When they speak of their experiences there, they speak of the wonderful Filipinos they've met, the culture, and the humorous stories. They share happy memories. Some even retain their language skills and speak to me in my dialect, Tagalog.

I admire their spirit. That lively spirit they have and the love for people and life itself— never allowing evil to destroy their nature. I thank them, our brave veterans and soldiers of God.

They are the greatest generation that ever lived!

DEATH and DYING

I cherish the moments—no matter how brief—when I'm able to interact with my patient near the end of life.

Just twelve hours ago, we were having a lively conversation, this patient and me. He was a spirited gentleman, who loved attention, conversation, and company. He was a bit cantankerous at times because he wasn't feeling well, but he always expressed his appreciation for us.

He recognized my voice and reached out his hand when I went to his bedside to tell him I'm his nurse tonight. He's resting comfortably, surrounded by his loving family. We are providing hospice care to alleviate any suffering and to make the process of dying comfortable for him.

I'm honored to be his nurse and grateful to be sharing this very special moment with him and his family.

SHERLOCK HOLMES, MD

We have a Sherlock Holmes at MWMC. He is a fascinating MD who would rather rely on his brain cells and 3 x 5 index cards than an iPhone. He drives a Mercedes Benz that has Bluetooth capability, though he doesn't need it. The Bluetooth, that is.

He can remember the first, middle, and last name of ANYONE in his past, present, and known future in a given conversation. He can speak coherently at almost the speed of sound. He is extremely versed in everything—from history to medicine. He can extract an accurate answer to ANY question within seconds without having to google it.

He can diagnose an ailment merely by talking to you and looking at you.

Really. Wow!

DRUG OF CHOICE. NOT

We often get patients who overdose on Tylenol. Accidentally or, yes, often intentionally. If you want to harm yourself with the intention of killing yourself, I have to tell you Tylenol is not the drug of choice. I can recommend better drugs or ways, but that's beside the point. Tylenol overdose causes liver failure, a miserable existence if you live through it, and/or a very painful death.

My favorite MD says that an adult should only take a maximum dose of 3 grams (3,000 mg) of Tylenol per 24 hrs. When he orders Tylenol for a patient, he writes his parameters within those guidelines. There are also prescription pain meds with Tylenol in it, so make sure to read the labels and do the math.

WISH UPON A STAR

I just realized that the best food to eat when I'm up all night for my graveyard shift is steak. Steak does the body good! I also wish that I had a miracle wand to sweep over my patients to erase all of their sadness … even just for twenty-four hours. And in those twenty-four hours, realize that they have great potential to be upstanding citizens instead of the lost and tortured souls they are.

MY PASSION

One of the best compliments I've ever received from a colleague: "I'm not worried when you're around."

TRUTH: The single most important reason I have enjoyed my career in nursing is the people I work with.

SMILE

Patient: "I want to go home tonight."

SK: "I'm afraid you're stuck with me tonight." The patient was silent, so I added, "I may not be the best company, but I'm the safest."

I got unanimous approval from his family who were at his bedside. And the patient managed a smile.

PATIENT CARE

It's really neat to see nursing as a choice of career for many of my friends. A lot of them make wonderful nurses! To those who are still in school, I have the utmost confidence that you will make wonderful nurses as well.

My long career as a registered nurse has been very rewarding. I've had my share of frustrations also, but mostly rewarding. I've said it before and I will say it again: I'm a diehard patient advocate. The number one duty of an RN is *patient safety*. I work really hard for the next part, but it's a must if you want to implement your duty. Leave your biases out of sight once you assume care of patients. Never fear to stand up for what is right. Always remain professional and stick to your convictions.

The worst thing a nurse can do is to watch a patient suffer or compromise a patient's safety because you didn't speak up. Another skill a good nurse should have is to always "anticipate the worst" so you can be prepared. Your critical-thinking and assessment skills come into play.

I have traveled all over the country and have worked with many physicians and healthcare personnel. The common denominator we all have as healthcare professionals is *patient safety*. I love all of my friends and colleagues who dedicate themselves to unwavering patient care.

ROMANTIC HEATHEN

SK: "I heard you've been married sixty-three years! What's your secret to a long-lasting marriage?"

Male patient: "I did what I was told!"

SK: "Smart man! You must love her very much."

Male patient: "I sure do."

His face lit up every time he spoke about his wife. I had to choke back tears. I'm such a romantic. A heathen … but a romantic heathen nonetheless.

COMPLIMENTS GALORE

1. Hans has an interesting way of complimenting you. According to him, I'm not the progeny of people who ate from the carcasses of animals, I'm the progeny of people who stood up against wooly mammoths and hunted sabretooth tigers, LOL. For those of you who know him, you can truly appreciate what a "beautiful mind" he has.

2. My male patient was waking up nicely in PACU. When he opened his eyes to look at me, he said, "Don't slap me, but you're very pretty." I rewarded him with my most tantalizing smile and thanked him for the compliment. He said, "I may be old but I always appreciate a nice view." I thanked him once again and continued to have a pleasant conversation with him until I sent him back to the medical–surgical unit.

3. My lovely, elderly patient in PACU thanked me for everything I did for her. She thanked me for medicating her for pain, for keeping her warm with blankets right out of our blanket warmer, for giving her ice chips. She called me her angel of mercy. I thanked her for her kind words and her grateful heart.

I'm going to get in trouble for this … but I'll take my chances! Once upon a time, Dr. B and I were chatting about the low census in ICU. I told him that I applied for a PRN job at another facility in order to support my many hobbies and maintain my lifestyle.

I then proceeded to tell him that I have an alternative … a sugar daddy. He kind of blushed and looked shy. He must have thought I was hitting on him! OMG!

PS: I was just making a BOLD statement. Seriously, I wouldn't dare hit on my colleagues … especially Dr. B, right? People who know my type would surely agree. Kidding aside, I'm always professional in the workplace. I did not mean to make Dr. B blush. I swear to God.

SK RN TIPS

In light of recent events and behaviors I have observed, I feel compelled to share some of the things that have made me successful in my career.

1. Don't burn your bridges.

2. Follow the chain of command; always remain professional and courteous in your dealings.

3. Don't jump to conclusions.

4. Don't be a whiner.

5. Be a team player.

6. There will always be changes, so remain flexible and always have a backup plan.

7. Always keep in mind that your job is an "at-will employment." They might fire you at any time for any reason. Or no reason. Therefore, always strive to be your best and don't rub the wrong people!

SK RN MUSINGS

These are random thoughts of mine that make their appearance at any given time and place.

1. Bad-ass: Two negative words combined = positive. Bad-ass is a word of endearment in my world.

2. Stay healthy … wash your hands … & don't share body fluids if you're sick. That's an order!

3. If someone asks you how you're doing … you should never say, "fine."

FINE stands for:

F - Freaked out

I - Insecure

N - Neurotic

E - Emotional

I used to be fine … but now … I'm bad-ass. LOL.

4. I want to leave something behind when I die, carved into the hearts of those I left behind. I want my offspring and loved ones to share good stories about me. That's all.

5. If death should take you tonight … just know how much I cared. I was there for you in your darkest night.

6. He talked about me. He looked forward to seeing me. He called my name when delirium consumed him.

7. If you hear a voice within you say, "you can't have chocolate," then, by all means, eat the damn chocolate and that voice will be silenced.

DEAR STEPHANIE

Dear Stephanie,

"I would like to thank you on behalf of my entire family for your hard work, compassion, and care you showed while working with our father. You stayed by his side, tirelessly adjusting, tweaking, keeping him alive as long as you possibly could. Thank you so much for your hard work and compassion you gave to our father in his last moments. We truly see you and your coworkers as heroes. God bless you!"

(A letter from a very lovely family.)

I will remember this moment forever. It was one of the most challenging nights of my critical-care nursing career. We worked very, very hard to save him. Despite our most valiant efforts, we lost him. The cause of death was sepsis from the flu—the worst case I've ever seen.

May you rest in peace, dear one.

AFTERWORD

"As a nurse, we have the opportunity to heal the heart, mind, soul and body of our patient, their families and ourselves. They may forget your name, but they will never forget how you make them feel."

– <u>Maya Angelou</u>

Follow Stephanie Klipple on...

Facebook: https://www.facebook.com/sklipple

Twitter: https://twitter.com/StephanieOHM

Instagram: https://www.instagram.com/spicychika/

Made in United States
Troutdale, OR
03/18/2024

18563788R00043